Healing with God's Earthly Gifts: Natural and Herbal Remedies

Kate Tietje

Modern Alternative Mama

# Contents

**Introduction** ...................... 4

  A Note of Caution/Disclaimer ....... 6

  Herbal Remedies Aren't

  Always Safe ................................. 7

  My 10 Favorite Herbs ................... 8

  Types of Herbal Preparations ...... 10

  Where to Buy Equipment ............. 12

  Chart of Common

  Conditions and Remedies ............. 13

**Remedies** ...................... 15

**The Basics** ...................... 16

  Basic Salve ................................. 17

  Basic Tincture ........................... 18

  Detox Bath 1 .............................. 19

  Detox Bath 2 .............................. 20

  Multivitamin Tincture ................. 21

**Respiratory Ailments** ...... 23

  Cold Kicker Tea 1 ....................... 24

  Cold Kicker Tea 2 ....................... 25

  Respiratory Ailment Syrup ......... 26

  Honey-Infused Cough Syrup ....... 27

  Homemade Vapor Rub .............. 28

  Garlic-Mullein Oil ...................... 29

**Head and Stomach** ......... 30

  Anti-Nausea Lozenges ................. 31

  Anti-Everything Pills .................. 32

  Sore Muscle and

  Headache Salve ........................... 33

**Skin and Surface Remedies 34**

  Anti-Fungal Foot Cream ............. 35

  Sore Skin Salve ........................... 36

  Skin Tightening Lotion ............... 37

  Healing Postpartum Bath ........... 38

**Balance** ........................... 39

  Nourishing Hormone

  Balancing Tea ............................. 40

  Hypothyroid Tincture ................. 41

  Calm Down Tincture ................... 42

**Other** .............................. 43

  Teething Tincture ....................... 44

  Magnesium Lotion ...................... 45

  Liver Pills .................................. 46

*"Healing with God's Earthly Gifts: Natural and Herbal Remedies"* is a book from the Modern Alternative Mama collection. Other books in this collection:

- *Real Food Basics, 2nd Ed.*
- *Healthy Pregnancy Super Foods*
- *Against the Grain: Delicious Recipes for Whole Food and Grain-Free Diet*
- *Treat Yourself: Real Food Desserts*
- *Wholesome Comfort: Whole Foods to Warm and Nourish Your Family*
- *Breast to Bib: Modern Alternative Mama's Guide to Nourishing Your Baby*
- *Simply Summer*
- *A Practical Guide to Children's Health*

Cover Design by Casey Spitnale, www.hellovoom.com.

# Introduction

We haven't used any over-the-counter (OTC) or prescription medication in our home since 2008. That's right – 6 years now. It's not that we haven't been sick, or run across the occasional health issue. We have four small children, so we certainly have. And my husband's faced a number of health concerns related to poor choices, family history, and information he didn't have as a child and teen. We've certainly had our share of "need" for remedies.

Yet, we haven't used any mainstream medication. Why not? Because we've learned about herbal and natural remedies to treat our family at home.

You, too, can learn to treat many illnesses at home. Most minor, acute illnesses (like colds, flu, stomach viruses, the occasional bout of insomnia, teething) can be safely and effectively treated at home with these alternative remedies. There's no reason to rush off to the doctor every time you or your child aren't feeling quite right!

I believe in the power of moms. I believe that families can intelligently do their research and learn ways to help their families naturally. I believe that for most of the conditions listed above (and many similar ones), moms can help themselves and their little ones feel better, naturally.

We don't need to rely on pharmaceuticals. We don't need to use round after round of antibiotics for simple ear infections, sinus infections, and the like. We can learn to feel better at home!

As we've been on our journey towards using exclusively natural remedies, we've found that we get sick less often, and we recover faster. We know what to reach for when symptoms begin, and we know what to do in the mean time to keep ourselves feeling well and strong. This has been a major bonus for us! I used to dread the winter times because I knew that we would have our share of illness.

But, not so much anymore. In 2013 – 14, we've faced only a couple very mild illnesses. My older children, as babies (when we still did some mainstream remedies and didn't know as much about the natural lifestyle) had many colds in their first couple of years. I remember getting up with them every hour at night because they couldn't breathe well from being stuffy. We sat near steamy showers, we suctioned, we begged for them to feel better and sleep.

In contrast, my fourth baby has had only a few colds, and no nights where we had to sit up because he couldn't breathe. Colds are gone in just a couple of days, too.

I can't promise this will be your experience. But I do know that natural remedies are powerful, and generally safe. I know that I much prefer using them in my home and that we're healthier for it. I hope that you find the same.

# A Note of Caution/Disclaimer

*D*espite my strong belief in the safety and efficacy of natural remedies, I must warn you that I am not a medical professional, nor a certified herbalist. I'm a mom, like you, who has learned to treat her family naturally. I'm sharing what I've learned and what works for us.

If you have any health concerns, or any chronic conditions, please seek the advice of a qualified medical professional to help you diagnose or treat your conditions. Although some of the remedies in this book may help to manage the symptoms of a chronic condition, they are not intended to cure it and are not a substitute for professional advice or management.

This book is intended to be used for mild illnesses, and if you have an emergency, please put the book down and call your doctor or 911.

# Herbal Remedies Aren't Always Safe

Many people have the mistaken impression that "natural equals safe." While for many of the remedies I offer in this book, this is true, this is not *always* the case. Some herbs are incredibly potent and can have serious side effects if used improperly or by the wrong people. I will note contraindications, if any, on individual recipes. If you are pregnant or nursing, please talk to your doctor or midwife before using any remedy.

Please treat herbs and natural remedies with care. Natural does not mean safe all the time, for all people. In addition to certain herbs having strong effects, the herbs can interact with prescription medications, reducing or increasing their effectiveness. This may cause an unsafe reaction. If you are using any prescription medication, or have any health conditions (especially liver or kidney disease), talk to your doctor before using *any* remedy, no matter how safe it seems.

Herbs should be treated like medicine, and remedies should be used with caution.

For the vast majority of people, who do not have health concerns, most of these remedies will be safe and will not pose a problem. Always ask a doctor or certified herbalist if you are concerned.

# My 10 Favorite Herbs

There are literally hundreds of different herbs out there. In fact, many plants that you would consider weeds in your garden are actually potential herbal remedies!

It would take far longer than I have to tell you about *every* available herb out there – and I don't know about all of them anyway. Plus, nobody wants to spend a ton of money buying dozens of different herbs when a few will do.

What follows are my ten favorite herbs, including why I love them so much, what I use them for, and who shouldn't use them.

*Ginger:* Ginger is usually used as a kitchen spice. It's an incredibly safe herb with many different uses. Ginger is anti-inflammatory, so it's good for pain, muscle aches, and headaches. It helps promote clear breathing during sinus infections or colds. It's also anti-nausea and great for stomachaches, motion sickness, and morning sickness. Some research even says it is anti-cancer.

The only people who should not use it are those with clotting disorders or who are about to undergo surgery – it's a blood thinner.

*Turmeric:* Turmeric is another kitchen spice, common in Indian cooking. It's bright yellow with a sort of bitter, unique flavor (it's the prime ingredient in curry). Turmeric is anti-inflammatory and great for headaches, muscle aches, menstrual cramps, or any sort of general pain. It helps colds and flu as well, and is anti-nausea. (Ginger and turmeric are in the same family and used similarly.) Some research says this is anti-cancer, as well.

**Do not use if you are about to undergo surgery or have a clotting disorder.**

*Mullein:* Mullein is an excellent herb for respiratory illnesses. It helps fight colds and flu, as well as bronchitis, sinus infections, even pertussis. It's also useful for insomnia.

No known contraindications.

*Acerola:* Acerola berries are a super food. They're extremely high in vitamin C and are a potent anti-oxidant. They're great for colds or the start of any infections because of the vitamin C content.

**Do not use if you are allergic to latex, because cross-reactivity is possible.**

*Elderberry:* These are another super food. They're often eaten as pie or jam, but they're also a great cold and flu remedy! Studies have shown that they can shorten the duration and severity of colds and flu and that they boost the immune system in general.

Do not use if you have an autoimmune condition – they boost the immune system so strongly that there's a tiny chance they can cause a "cytokine storm" which can result in more severe illness or even death. (This side effect is theoretical and has never actually been reported.)

*Catnip:* Yes, catnip – the same stuff that makes cats crazy. In humans, though, it produces relaxation and helps people to sleep. It's also useful for digestive upset, skin conditions, and respiratory infections.

**Do not use if you are pregnant or breastfeeding.** Catnip is in the mint family, which can bring on menstruation and may reduce milk supply. (Many women do use catnip in small amounts while nursing with no problems.)

*Yarrow:* This herb is very useful for wounds and bleeding. It can help to stop bleeding both internally and externally. It's anti-inflammatory, it helps to increase sweat and reduce fevers. Yarrow can be used topically or internally, and even to reduce menstrual cramps and excessive bleeding during periods.

**Do not use if you are pregnant, because yarrow can bring on menstruation**.

*Arnica:* This herb is excellent for muscle pain and soreness. It can relieve headaches, reduce muscle cramps and tension (including afterpains from childbirth), and soothe sunburns. It may help reduce bruising and speed healing time when used on wounds.

Do not use internally.

*Cloves:* A simple cooking spice, cloves have powerful medicinal properties too. The most common use for cloves is to aid oral pain – both in adults, and in teething babies. They reduce inflammation and may relieve infections too.

Do not use if you have a bleeding disorder or about to undergo surgery, because clove can interfere with clotting.

# Types of Herbal Preparations

There are several different methods of preparing herbs to use as remedies. Before we get to the actual remedies, I want to explain the different preparations, how to create them, and when to use them.

## Teas

Preparing herbs as a tea is probably the most common way to use them. This is simple, and involves using a small amount of herbs (usually 1 – 2 tsp. per cup of water), steeped in boiling water for a short time (5 – 10 minutes). This preparation is a good way to get nourishment from herbs (vitamins and minerals) as well as help with minor ailments, like colds.

It's also safe for children and, in some cases, babies, because of the comparatively weak effects that a tea brings. Plus, it requires no special equipment – just a way to heat the water and strain the herb out of the tea after it's brewed.

## Infusions

An infusion is similar to a tea – it's water-based – but it's much, much stronger. An infusion is usually brewed from 1 oz. of dry herbs (by weight) in 2 – 4 cups of boiling water, steeped for quite awhile (1 hour to overnight). An infusion is recommended for nourishing and adaptogenic herbs to gain the most benefit from them. Pregnancy teas would be an example of herbs typically consumed in an infusion.

It's best not to use this for an herb with potent effects, because the dose could easily be too large. It is probably not best for children either.

## Tinctures

A tincture is a method of both preserving herbs and extracting their medicinal qualities. Tinctures are prepared with fresh or dried herbs and alcohol (usually vodka), vegetable glycerin, or vinegar. A large amount of herbs is steeped in the tincturing medium usually for 6 weeks, until the liquid has become dark brown and full of the herb's medicinal qualities. The tincture is typically strained at that point, and is good for several months to several years. Small doses are needed, sometimes as little as a few drops, or up to a couple tablespoons (for nourishing tinctures).

Tinctures can be appropriate for anyone, depending on herb and dose.

## Pills

Capsules of herbs are another simple way to benefit. Many people who buy herbal supplements get dried, sometimes powdered herbs in capsules from health food stores. The advantages are that these are simple to buy or to make and easy (for most) to take. The dose can also be somewhat standardized.

The downside is that they're not that potent (herbs are bulky) and some can't swallow pills. This method is best for more potent herbs, used on an irregular basis.

## Salves

Sometimes, herbs are needed topically. While it's possible to use a cloth soaked with tea or infusion, a simpler method is often to use a salve. A salve is an oil that is infused with an herb or combination of herbs, then combined with beeswax to make a solid cream. It's rubbed into affected areas as needed. Salves are for external use only, and are usually safe for anyone.

## Poultices

Poultices are less common now than they used to be, but are still used. A poultice is usually an herb (often a root, like an onion, ginger, turmeric, etc.) that is heated gently and chopped and sweated to release the juices. This herb and the juices are poured, still very warm, onto a cloth and wrapped up and placed on an affected area. Poultices are often used to loosen congestion in the chest, for example. These are safe for most (as long as they aren't too hot).

# Where to Buy Equipment

If you're planning to prepare herbal remedies, you will need some basic equipment. Exactly what you need will depend on which remedies you intend to make. These are the most common items.

*Glass jars:* Jars are used for so many things. I like to use mason jars, because they are inexpensive and available anywhere. Jars will be used for making teas and infusions, creating and storing tinctures, storing lotions, storing dry herbs, and more. Get a variety of sizes, although I use the pint and quart ones most often. Smaller jars are better for lotions or salves.

*Brown glass bottles:* Tinctures are ideally stored in these bottles. I choose ½ oz. bottles so that they will travel well.

*Cheesecloth:* I actually use birdseye cotton (the type that is used in cloth diapers). You'll find this at cooking stores or fabric stores. I like to keep several pieces of it around so that I always have one clean and ready to use. Buy a couple of yards of fabric (any smooth, non-fuzzy fabric will do) and cut into 12x12 rectangles.

*Herbs:* I buy mine from Mountain Rose Herbs online. They are largely wild-crafted or organically grown. Sometimes local health food stores will carry them as well.

*Capsules:* I buy mine on Amazon, NOW brand. They also carry them at some health food stores.

*Glycerin:* I buy NOW brand on Amazon. Some types are made from palm or coconut; others may be made from corn or soy, so read the labels.

*Oils and Butters:* These are available from Mountain Rose Herbs, as well as health food stores, Amazon, and various online soap- and lotion-making stores.

*Raw honey:* This is best purchased from a farmer or beekeeper near you.

*Essential Oils:* There are a number of good places to purchase these. There are some on Amazon, there is Heritage Essential Oils, and there is doTERRA. This could turn into a topic in and of itself (where is the best place to buy) so I'll let you choose what you prefer.

*Other:* Most other items can be purchased on Amazon or at your local health food store.

# Chart of Common Conditions and Remedies

| Condition | Remedy |
| --- | --- |
| **Cough** | Detox Bath 1 or 2, Honey-Infused Cough Syrup, Cold Kicker Tea 1 or 2, Homemade Vapor Rub |
| **Cold** | Detox Bath 1 or 2, Cold Kicker Tea 1 or 2, Respiratory Ailment Syrup |
| **Ear Infection** | Garlic-Mullein Oil, Anti-Everything Pills, Detox Bath 1 or 2, Cold Kicker Tea 1 or 2 |
| **Sore Throat** | Cold Kicker Tea 1 or 2, Anti-Everything Pills |
| **Sinus Infection** | Cold Kicker Tea 1 or 2, Anti-Everything Pills, Respiratory Ailment Syrup, Neti pot, Homemade Vapor Rub |
| **Stomachache** | Cold Kicker Tea 1, Anti-Nausea Lozenges |
| **Nausea/ Vomiting** | Bentonite clay capsules, activated charcoal, Anti-Nausea Lozenges, Anti-Everything Pills |
| **Bronchitis** | Cold Kicker Tea 2, Respiratory Ailment Syrup |
| **Headache** | Sore Muscle and Headache Salve, Anti-Everything Pills, Magnesium Lotion |
| **Migraine** | Sore Muscle and Headache Salve, Anti-Everything Pills, Magnesium Lotion, Lavender or Peppermint essential oil |
| **Pertussis** | Respiratory Ailment Syrup, Anti-Everything Pills, Honey-Infused Cough Syrup, Detox Bath 1 or 2 |
| **Flu** | Anti-Everything Pills, Respiratory Ailment Syrup, Cold Kicker Tea 1 or 2, Detox Bath 1 or 2 |
| **Strep Throat** | Anti-Everything Pills, Cold Kicker Tea 2, Detox Bath 2, Respiratory Ailment Syrup |
| **ADHD** | Calm Down Tincture, Magnesium Lotion, fish oil |
| **Anxiety** | Calm Down Tincture, Magnesium Lotion, Hormone Balancing Tea |
| **Fatigue** | Magnesium Lotion, Liver Pills |
| **Growing Pains** | Magnesium Lotion |
| **Insomnia** | Magnesium Lotion, Calm Down Tincture |
| **Menstrual Cramps** | Anti-Everything Pills, Detox Bath 2, Hormone Balancing Tea |

| Condition | Remedy |
| --- | --- |
| *Hypothyroid* | Hypothyroid Tincture, Liver Pills, Magnesium Lotion |
| *Yeast Infections* | Anti-Everything Pills, Anti-Fungal Cream |
| *Asthma* | Lobelia tincture, Magnesium Lotion |
| *Food Allergies* | Probiotics, Magnesium Lotion, Detox Bath 1 or 2 |
| *Eczema* | Skin Soothing Lotion, Magnesium Lotion, probiotics |
| *Grumpy/Fussy Children* | Calm Down Tincture, Magnesium Lotion |
| *Teething* | Teething Tincture |
| *Split Skin* | Skin Soothing Lotion, bentonite clay mask |
| *Diaper rash* | Skin Soothing Lotion, bentonite clay mask |
| *Diarrhea* | Dandelion leaf or root tea, Multi-Vitamin Tincture |
| *Constipation* | Magnesium Lotion, Hypothyroid Tincture |
| *Depression* | Hormone Balancing Tea, Magnesium Lotion, fish oil |
| *Chicken Pox* | Skin Soothing Lotion, Detox Bath 1 or 2 |
| *Fever* | Detox Bath 1 or 2, yarrow tea |
| *Poison Ivy* | Skin Soothing Lotion, bentonite clay cream, jewelweed or plantain salve |
| *Postpartum Soreness* | Postpartum Herbal Bath, Hormone Balancing Tea |
| *Dehydration (minor)* | Cold Kicker Tea 1 (add a pinch of sea salt) |
| *Morning Sickness* | Col Kicker Tea 1, Magnesium Lotion, Ginger or fennel tincture |
| *Tonsillitis* | Respiratory Ailment Syrup, Cold Kicker Tea 1 or 2, Detox Bath 1 or 2 |
| *Excessive Bleeding* | Shepherd's purse or yarrow salve or tincture |
| *Preterm Labor* | Magnesium Lotion |
| *Unbalanced Blood Sugar* | Magnesium Lotion, probiotics |
| *Low Milk Supply* | Liver Pills, Hormone Balancing Tea, fenugreek, blessed thistle |

# Remedies

# The Basics

# Basic Salve

*I*t would be impossible to list every single possible salve in this book. Instead, if there's a salve that you want to use but it isn't in here, use the chart of remedies and these basic instructions to create your own.

## Ingredients:

- ¼ c. dried herbs (can be one herb or a combination)
- ½ c. liquid oil (olive, apricot, etc.)
- 2 tbsp. beeswax
- 20 – 30 drops essential oils*

*Optional

*Step 1:* Heat the oil gently until warm, but not hot. Remove from heat.

*Step 2:* Add the dried herbs to the oil, and allow them to steep for 20 – 30 minutes.

*Step 3:* Pour the oil through a piece of cheesecloth and squeeze out all the oil.

*Step 4:* Heat the oil again (just very warm, not hot) and add the beeswax until melted.

*Step 5:* Pour into a 4-oz. jar.

*Step 6:* Allow to cool for 10 – 15 minutes, then add essential oils, if using, and stir gently.

*Step 7:* Allow to cool completely before using.

*Use:* Spread a small amount of salve on affected area as needed. Lasts 6 – 12 months.

*Caution:* For external use only. Additional cautions depend on which herbs are used.

# Basic Tincture

*I*t is also not possible to offer recipes for every possible tincture out there. Be sure to consult an herbalist or do your own research if you're not sure which herb(s) to use. Single herb tinctures are simplest, but multi-herb tinctures can be created depending on your needs.

There are two basic tinctures that you can use. Alcohol-based tinctures are best for occasional medicinal uses (they will extract most potently and last the longest), and glycerin tinctures are best for frequent use or small children.

## Alcohol Tincture

It's easiest to use 100-proof here, because most tinctures are half water and half alcohol. 100 proof is exactly that, so no measuring or guessing needed.

### Ingredients:

- 100-proof vodka
- Herbs of choice (fresh if possible)

*Step 1:* Add herbs to a quart-sized mason jar. Fill near the top with fresh, or about half full with dried.

*Step 2:* Fill the jar with alcohol.

*Step 3:* Cap the jar, shake to combine, and label with the type and date. Allow it to sit in a dark place for 6 weeks.

*Step 4:* Strain the herbs through a piece of cheesecloth, squeezing to get all the liquid out.

*Step 5:* Store in a brown glass bottle, labeled.

## Glycerin Tincture

### Ingredients:

- Vegetable glycerin
- Filtered water
- Herbs of choice

Use equal amounts of glycerin and water. Follow the instructions for alcohol tincture, above, using glycerin and water instead of alcohol.

*Use:* Take 2 – 10 drops as needed (for medicinal tinctures) and 1 tsp. to 2 tbsp. (for nourishing tinctures) daily. Alcohol lasts 2 – 3 years; glycerin lasts 6 – 12 months.

*Caution:* Depends on the chosen herbs. Read the individual cautions carefully.

# Detox Bath 1

This simple detox bath helps to pull junk out through the skin. It's excellent after exercise or a massage, or just as a general "upkeep." It's fairly gentle and safe for children.

## Ingredients:

- ½ c. bath salts (we like Redmond Bath Salts)
- ½ c. baking soda

*Step 1:* Add both ingredients to a very warm or hot bath; stir to dissolve.

*Step 2:* Soak for 20 – 30 minutes.

*Use:* Take a bath 2 – 3 times per week, or as needed. Dry ingredients last 1 – 2 years.

*Caution:* Do not take a very hot bath if pregnant. Stand up slowly after bathing; this may make you dizzy.

# Detox Bath 2

This detox bath is a little bit stronger. It's better used if there is a greater need to detox in general (for adults) or in times of illness. It can be used for children, but reduce the amounts by half and soak for less time.

## Ingredients:

- ½ c. bentonite clay
- ½ c. bath salts

*Step 1:* Add both ingredients to a very warm or hot bath (as hot as possible for adults); stir to dissolve.

*Step 2:* Soak for 20 – 30 minutes.

*Use:* Take a bath daily during a cleanse or when beginning the GAPS diet, or as needed during illness. Dry ingredients last 1 – 2 years.

*Caution:* Do not use if you are pregnant. Stand up slowly after bathing; this may make you dizzy. Be careful if breastfeeding, as toxins will get into your lymphatic system and pass into your milk.

# Multivitamin Tincture

Many people are seeking healthy multivitamins. A lot of the options on the market aren't necessarily good for you – which is why I came up with this solution: a homemade herbal version!

These herbs **are extremely rich in nutrients, and since they're plants, these nutrients are in a balanced, synergistic form.** Adaptogenic herbs are known to help balance and help the body gently, without any side effects (which some herbs *can* have). These herbs are safe to take daily, and are well-absorbed by the body.

- Alfalfa is rich in vitamin K, C, and E; iron, calcium, magnesium, phosphorus, sulfur, chlorine, sodium, potassium, and silicon.
- Dandelion leaf is rich in vitamins A, C, D, and B complex as well as iron, magnesium, zinc, potassium, manganese, copper, choline, calcium, boron, and silicon.
- Catnip is rich in manganese, folic acid, phosphorous, sodium, sulphur, pantothenic acid, vitamin A and vitamin B-complex.
- Nettles are rich in calcium, magnesium, iron, potassium, phosphorous, manganese, silica, iodine, silicon, sodium, sulfur, vitamin C, beta-carotene, and B complex vitamins.
- Spearmint is rich in vitamins A, B-complex, and C, plus iron and manganese.

For best results, take it with fermented cod liver oil, so that the fat-soluble vitamins will be properly absorbed.

## Ingredients:

- 6 tbsp. alfalfa
- 6 tbsp. dandelion
- 3 tbsp. catnip*
- 3 tbsp. nettle
- 1.5 tbsp. spearmint*
- 2 c. vegetable glycerin
- 2 c. filtered water

*These are in the mint family, which should be used with caution during pregnancy. Some say, best avoided. However, I used it during pregnancy with no issues. Use your judgment, and swap them for an equal amount of dried nettles if you have any cause for concern.

*Step 1:* Add all of the dried herbs to a quart-sized glass jar.

*Step 2:* Add the glycerin and water.

*Step 3:* Add a lid and shake gently to combine.

*Step 4:* Allow to sit for six weeks in a dark place, or use the crockpot method that takes 2 – 3 days.

*Step 5:* Strain through a clean dish towel, squeezing to get all the liquid out.

*Step 6:* Store in a glass jar in a cool, dark place.

*Use:* Take 1 tsp. for children and 1 tbsp. for adults (up to 2 – 3 tbsp. for pregnant and nursing women) per day.  Use your judgment and take what "feels right" to you as an adult – you can't overdose on this.  Lasts 6 – 12 months.

*Caution:* Pregnant women should be careful with catnip and spearmint.  Do not use alfalfa if you have lupus or a clotting disorder.

# Respiratory Ailments

# Cold Kicker Tea 1

T his cold-kicker tea is very simple and the ingredients are available in any grocery store!  Use as often as desired.  2 – 3 cups a day is fine, and especially before bed-time.

## Ingredients:

- 3 – 4 thin slices of fresh ginger
- 2 c. filtered water
- Juice of ½ lemon
- 1 – 2 tsp. raw honey

*Step 1:* Add the water to a medium saucepan with the ginger slices.

*Step 2:* Boil the ginger for 10 minutes, until the tea is golden-colored.  Remove from heat and remove ginger slices.

*Step 3:* Pour into a mug and add lemon juice and raw honey to taste.  Drink while hot.

*Use:* Drink immediately.  Lasts 3 – 6hours.

*Caution:* Ginger should not be used by those with bleeding disorders or who are about to undergo surgery.

# Cold Kicker Tea 2

This tea has some less-easy-to-find herbs, but it's great if you have a more serious cold or sinus infection (or even bronchitis or possibly pertussis – see a doctor if you have serious symptoms like trouble breathing, though). It's a stronger remedy but helps to clear up sinuses, soothe sore throats, and aid rest.

## Ingredients:

- 1 tbsp. mullein leaves
- 1 tsp. fenugreek seeds
- 1 c. water
- Raw honey to taste

*Step 1:* Combine mullein, fenugreek, and water in a saucepan.

*Step 2:* Boil for 5 minutes, then allow to steep, removed from the heat, for 15 – 20 minutes.

*Step 3:* Strain out the herbs through a sieve or piece of cheesecloth.

*Step 4:* Sweeten to taste and serve very warm.

*Use:* Drink immediately or refrigerate for 1 – 2 days.

*Caution:* Fenugreek should not be used during pregnancy.

# Respiratory Ailment Syrup

When my eight-month-old got a bad cold right before the holidays, I knew I had to create something good to kick it quick. I combined my best respiratory herbs to make this syrup. I took the syrup myself as a breastfeeding mom, and it kicked his cold in just two days!

It's some pretty awesome stuff and can likely be used for a sinus infection, flu, bronchitis, or any respiratory illness that isn't responding to some of the more mundane cold teas. (As always, see a doctor for serious symptoms, like trouble breathing.)

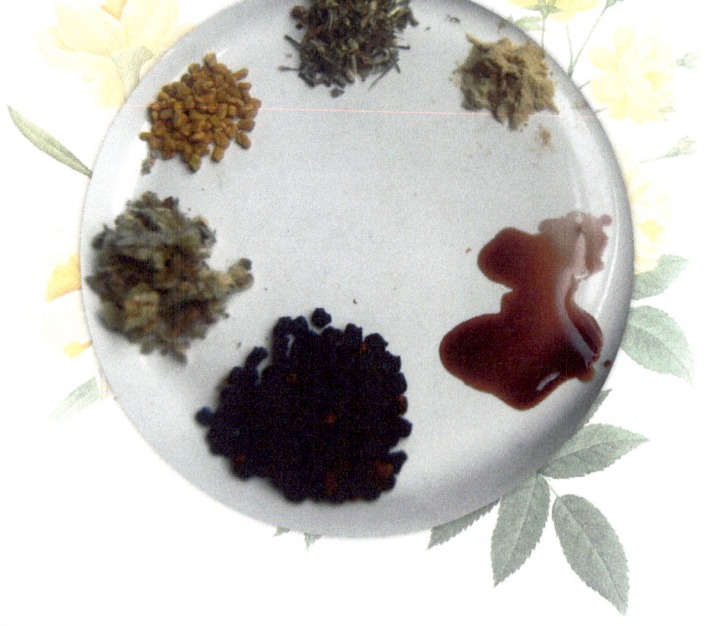

## Ingredients:

- 1 c. elderberries
- 1/2 c. mullein leaves
- 1 tbsp. fenugreek seeds
- 3 tbsp. yarrow leaf
- 2 c. filtered water
- 3/4 c. raw honey
- 1/4 c. acerola powder

*Step 1:* Combine the elderberries, mullein, fenugreek, yarrow, and water in a medium saucepan.

*Step 2:* Boil the herbs for about 5 minutes, then remove from the heat.

*Step 3:* Allow to steep for 20 – 30 minutes.

*Step 4:* Strain through a clean dish towel and discard the herbs.

*Step 5:* Add the raw honey and acerola powder to the liquid and stir until dissolved.

*Step 6:* Refrigerate when not using for up to a month.

*Use:* Take 1 tsp. for kids or 1 tbsp. for adults every 1 – 4 hours at the onset of symptoms (for one to two days), then take 1 – 2 times per day until symptoms disappear. Lasts 1 month.

*Caution:* Fenugreek and yarrow should not be used during pregnancy. Use elderberry with care if you have an autoimmune condition. Do not give raw honey to babies under 1 year.

# Honey-Infused Cough Syrup

I s a cough keeping you up at night? This simple infused honey syrup uses the raw honey that's been shown to safely quiet coughs, *plus* additional herbs to help combat the cold that's causing it. It tastes great, too, so most people won't complain about taking it!

## Ingredients:

- 1 c. raw honey
- ¼ c. mullein leaves
- ¼ c. wild cherry bark
- 1 tbsp. slippery elm bark

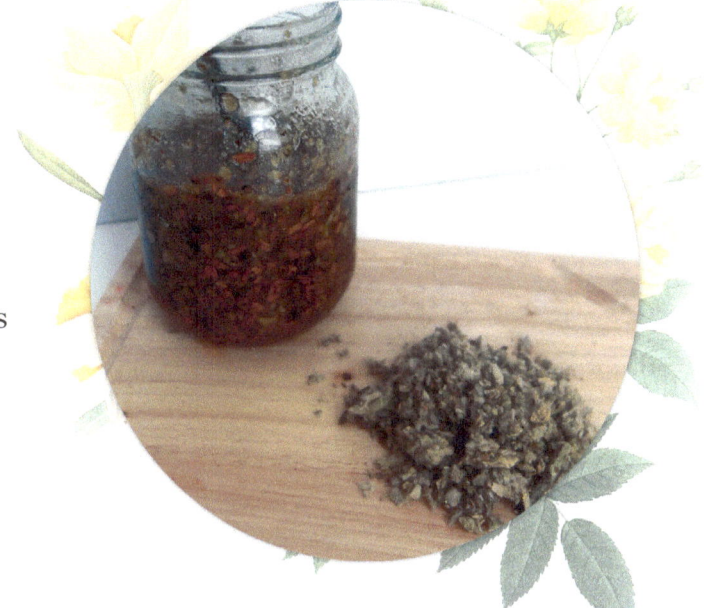

*Step 1:* Add the honey to a glass jar (pint sized or larger).

*Step 2:* Add the herbs and stir them up.

*Step 3:* Allow this to sit in a dark place for 3 – 6 weeks.

*Step 4:* Pour the mixture into a saucepan and create a double boiler – pan underneath filled with water.

*Step 5:* Very gently heat the honey mixture just until it's thin enough to strain.

*Step 6:* Strain through a clean dishtowel or a piece of cheesecloth to remove the herbs.

*Step 7:* Pour the infused honey into a clean jar and keep in a cool, dry place.

*Use:* Take one spoonful as needed, especially before bed. Lasts 1 – 2 years.

*Caution:* Do not give raw honey to babies under 1 year.

# Homemade Vapor Rub

Simple vapor rubs can promote clear breathing and restful sleep when someone is coughing or stuffed up. Commercial products similar to this are based on petroleum jelly, which is not safe for the skin. This version is very safe, even for younger babies, and also very effective.

## Ingredients:

- 5 tbsp. extra virgin coconut oil
- 1 tbsp. olive oil
- 2 tbsp. beeswax
- 8 – 10 drops tea tree essential oil
- 15 – 20 drops rosemary essential oil

*Step 1:* In a small pan over low heat, melt the coconut oil and olive oil.

*Step 2:* Add the beeswax, chopped up or in granules (mine was in a large chunk, so I chopped) and stir until melted.

*Step 3:* Add the essential oils and stir to combine.

*Step 4:* Pour into a 4-oz. glass jar and allow to cool. This mix is not completely solid even when cool, so be careful of that when you open the jar.

*Use:* Before bed, put this mixture on the *feet* and then put socks over it. When it's put on the feet, it's absorbed quickly into the body and it goes through the whole system. Lasts 3 – 6 months.

*Caution:* For external use only.

# Garlic-Mullein Oil

For earaches, nothing beats this simple oil. It's quick to prepare, and it soothes sore ears quickly and easily. We've taken care of ear infections in a matter of hours with this!

## Ingredients:

- 1/2 c. coconut oil
- 2 cloves garlic, crushed
- 2 tbsp. mullein leaves

*Step 1:* Combine all ingredients in a small saucepan.

*Step 2:* Heat very gently on low heat, just for a minute or two (the oil needs to be warm, but not hot).

*Step 3:* Allow the oil to sit for 5 – 10 minutes off the heat.

*Step 4:* Strain through a piece of cheesecloth (you don't want any of the herbs to get in the ear).

*Step 5:* Pour into a glass jar for storage.

*Use:* Pour a small amount, about ¼ tsp. into the affected ear while lying on your side. If solidified, scoop up a small amount and allow it to melt in the ear. Gently tug on the earlobe to allow it to move down inside. Let the oil sit for 5 minutes, then sit up and allow it to drain out. Lasts 2 – 3 days.

*Caution:* Do not use if ear drum has burst, or if there is any bleeding or pus draining from the ear.

# Head and Stomach

# Anti-Nausea Lozenges

*I*f your tummy's not feeling quite right, sucking on one of these will help it feel better fast. This combination of herbs is great for any stomach upset – indigestion, morning sickness, motion sickness, etc.

## Ingredients:

- 4 - 5 slices ginger
- 3 tbsp. fennel
- 2 tbsp. chamomile
- 2 tbsp. lemon balm
- 1 c. water + extra
- 1 c. cane sugar

**Step 1:** Combine ginger, fennel, chamomile, lemon balm, and water in a saucepan.

**Step 2:** Boil for 10 minutes, then remove from heat.

**Step 3:** Allow this "tea" to steep for 30 minutes, then strain through a clean dish towel.

**Step 4:** Measure the "tea" and add additional water as needed to make 1 c. total.

**Step 5:** Pour the "tea" into a clean saucepan and stir in the cane sugar.

**Step 6:** Boil until the "hard crack" stage is reached; 300 – 310 degrees.

**Step 7:** While the syrup is boiling, prepare a cookie sheet by covering with parchment paper OR prepare candy molds.

**Step 8:** When the syrup is finished, quickly pour it onto the parchment paper or into molds. (If you wait more than a minute or two, it will solidify into hard candy in the pan.)

**Step 9:** Allow the lozenges to harden, then pop them out or use a sharp knife to break them up (from parchment paper) and store in a cool, dry place – a bag or glass jar in a pantry.

**Use:** Take 1 as needed for upset stomach. Lasts 3 – 6 months.

**Caution:** Do not use ginger if you have a bleeding disorder or are undergoing surgery soon. Chamomile may cause allergic reactions.

# Anti-Everything Pills

*I* really don't know how you'd describe these pills, exactly. They are a combination of three powerful herbs, which can fight just about any type of virus, bacteria, inflammation, pain, infection...you name it. Hence, "anti-everything."

They contain turmeric, which is strongly anti-inflammatory, anti-cancer, and all around awesome. Also acerola berry powder (pure), which is very high in vitamin C. Finally, goldenseal root powder, which is anti-bacterial, anti-fungal, anti-viral, immune-boosting, and enhances the potency of other herbs it's taken with.

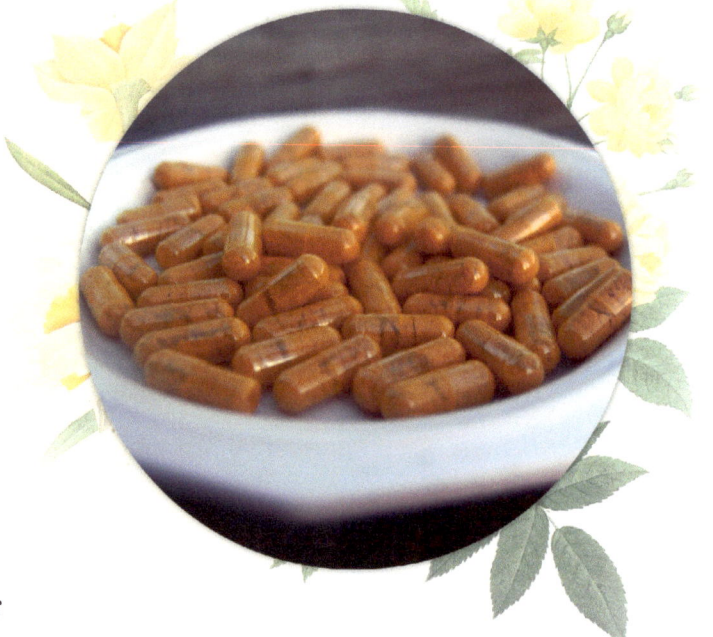

If you are primarily interested in the anti-inflammatory action and wish to take these pills daily, either use plain turmeric, or turmeric and acerola. Do not include goldenseal for daily use.

The ingredients below are measured by *weight*, not volume!

## Ingredients:

- 3 oz. turmeric root powder
- 1 1/2 oz. acerola berry powder
- 1/2 oz. goldenseal root powder
- 500 "00" gelatin capsules

*Step 1:* Weigh each herb carefully, using a kitchen scale.

*Step 2:* Combine all the herbs in a glass jar, then cap the jar and gently shake to combine.

*Step 3:* Use a capsule machine to fill the capsules easily, OR take them apart, fill the larger side, and top with the smaller side. (Capsule makers are inexpensive at around $12 and *much* faster.)

*Step 4:* Store the finished pills in a glass jar (500 will fill about 1 quart jar).

*Use:* Take 1 – 2 as needed, for headaches, muscle aches, menstrual cramps, sore throat, feeling of oncoming illness, etc. Lasts 1 year.

*Caution:* Do not use daily. People with bleeding disorders or who are about to undergo surgery should not use turmeric.

# Sore Muscle and Headache Salve

This simple salve is wonderful for many types of skin and muscle pain. It helps relieve muscle tension and soothe the headaches. We've even used it successfully on sunburns. It's one of the remedies I make sure to bring when we're traveling because of its many uses.

## Ingredients:

- 1/2 c. avocado oil*
- 1 tbsp. lavender flowers
- 1 tbsp. yarrow
- 1 tbsp. arnica flowers
- 2 tbsp. bees wax

*May use jojoba, sweet almond, olive, or other liquid oil

*Step 1:* In a small saucepan, combine the herbs and oil.

*Step 2:* Create a double boiler by placing this pot in a larger pot filled with water.

*Step 3:* Turn the pot on low-medium heat and allow it to heat the oil very gently. Simmer (don't allow the oil to cook the herbs) for 20 – 30 minutes.

*Step 4:* Strain the oil through a clean dish towel.

*Step 5:* Clean the pot to get rid of the herb residue, then return the oil to the clean, dry pot.

*Step 6:* Add the beeswax and heat on low until melted.

*Step 7:* Pour into a small glass jar and allow to cool.

*Use:* Rub a small amount onto sore skin or into sore muscles as needed. Lasts 6 – 12 months.

*Caution:* For external use only.

# Skin and Surface Remedies

# Anti-Fungal Foot Cream

*I*f you've been struggling with athlete's foot or another type of fungal infection, this is a natural remedy that can help to banish the fungus. Combined with a low-sugar diet, it may remove the fungus in a matter of days or weeks!

This fungal cream may also be beneficial for warts or yeast infections elsewhere on the skin.

## Ingredients:

- 7 tbsp. extra virgin organic coconut oil
- 40 drops Grapefruit Seed Extract
- 15 drops tea tree oil
- 4 oz. glass jar

*Step 1:* In a double boiler over low heat, melt the coconut oil.

*Step 2:* Add the GSE and TTO and stir together to combine.

*Step 3:* Pour the mixture into the glass jar and let it cool completely.

*Use:* Apply as needed to skin suffering from any type of fungal infection, including yeast infection (please don't apply directly to any internal parts; if you have yeast-like rashes on your arms or legs though, apply there!). Lasts 6 – 12 months.

*Caution:* For external use only.

# Sore Skin Salve

This simple salve can be used for diaper rash, eczema, or any other type of "sore skin" out there.  It's safe with cloth diapers, too.

## Ingredients:

- 1 tbsp. calendula flowers
- 1 tbsp. chamomile flowers
- 1 tbsp. lavender buds
- 1 tsp. comfrey leaves
- 3 oz. olive oil
- 2 tbsp. bees wax

*Step 1:* In a double boiler, combine the herbs and olive oil.

*Step 2:* Over low heat, allow the herbs to infuse for 20 – 30 minutes.  Do not let it get too hot and 'fry' the herbs.

*Step 3:* Strain the oil through a piece of cheesecloth, squeezing it all out.

*Step 4:* In a clean saucepan, combine the oil and beeswax over low heat, until the wax is melted.

*Step 5:* Pour into a 4-oz. glass jar.  Allow to cool completely before use.

*Use:* Spread a small amount on affected area as needed.  Lasts 6 – 12 months.

*Caution:* For external use only.  Do not use if allergic to ragweed.

# Skin Tightening Lotion

T his one actually came about for two reasons. First, I had noticed that when I had been applying my magnesium lotion to my abdomen, my stretch marks were disappearing. That was kind of cool. Second, some family members had recently lost a lot of weight and were looking for a natural, homemade formula to tighten up extra skin. Some research led to this cream.

It will help to tighten up loose skin, smooth skin, reduce cellulite, and reduce wrinkles and stretch marks. Try it anywhere you need a little "rejuvenation." If you want to use it on your face, use pure water instead of magnesium oil.

## Ingredients:

- 2 oz. apricot kernel oil
- 2 tsp. dried rosemary
- 2 tsp. dried sage
- 2 oz. magnesium oil (1 oz. water + 2 oz. magnesium chloride flakes)
- 15 drops frankincense essential oil
- 15 drops lavender essential oil
- 10 drops grapefruit essential oil
- 2 tbsp. beeswax

*Step 1:* In a double boiler, add apricot oil, rosemary, and sage. Heat on low for 20 – 30 minutes.

*Step 2:* Strain the oil through a piece of cheesecloth, squeezing out all the oil.

*Step 3:* Heat 1 oz. water until warm, then dissolve the magnesium chloride flakes in it. Measure out ¼ c. total to use for this recipe.

*Step 4:* Heat the infused apricot oil in a clean pan on low heat. Add the beeswax and allow it to melt.

*Step 5:* Combine the oil and magnesium solution in a blender. Add the essential oils.

*Step 6:* Whip on medium to high speed until thick and white.

*Step 7:* Quickly pour into a 4-oz. glass jar, scraping with a spatula if needed.

*Use:* Spread a small amount on affected skin daily. Lasts 3 – 6 months.

*Caution:* For external use only.

# Healing Postpartum Bath

After birth, it's not uncommon at all to be rather sore for awhile – especially if you've torn and had stitches. This soothing herbal bath can help you to heal more quickly and have less pain.

## Ingredients:

- ½ c. yarrow
- 1 c. comfrey leaves
- ½ c. uva ursi
- ½ c. calendula
- 1 c. lavender flowers

*Step 1:* Mix all herbs together and store in a glass jar.

*Use:* Place one handful (about ½ c.) of herbs in a muslin bag, and steep in boiling water for 20 minutes, then pour the water into a bath (comfortable temperature). Add a handful of bath salts too. Dry herbs last 6 – 12 months.

*Caution:* For external use only.

# Balance

# Nourishing Hormone Balancing Tea

This tea is wonderful for postpartum, menstrual cramps or heavy periods, or other general hormonal imbalances. It isn't strong enough by itself to completely correct major issues, but it helps to gently balance the body. The herbs are what's known as adaptogenic, which means they nourish the body and correct imbalances without producing side effects.

## Ingredients:

- 1 c. dried nettles
- 1 c. red raspberry leaf
- ½ c. alfalfa
- ½ c. dandelion leaf
- ½ c. spearmint leaf

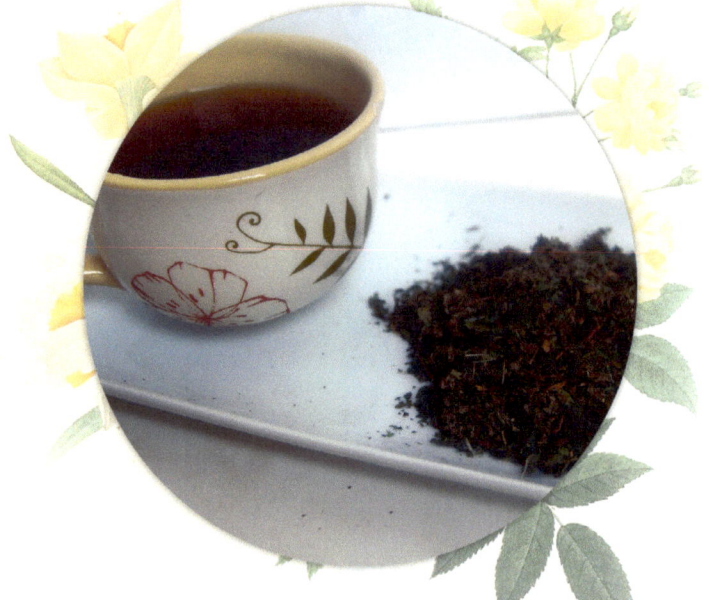

**Step 1:** Add all of the dry herbs to a large Ziploc-style bag.

**Step 2:** Seal the bag and shake to combine.

**Use:** Use a handful of the mix (about 1/3 c.) in 2 – 3 cups of hot water to make an infusion. Allow the infusion to steep for 30 – 60 minutes. Dry herbs last for about 1 year. Consume the tea within 6 hours or refrigerate for 1 – 2 days.

**Caution:** Do not use alfalfa if you have blood clots or lupus, because it causes blood to clot faster. Do not use spearmint leaf if you are pregnant and use caution if breastfeeding (it may lower milk supply).

# Hypothyroid Tincture

Hypothyroidism runs in our family, so I knew I needed something natural to combat it. I don't like the idea of synthetic or even bio-identical hormones because I think that they mess with the body's homeostasis (although they may be necessary for those with severe issues). Instead, I chose a blend of herbs that are known to help balance and nourish the thyroid gland.

Please note all the herb measurements below are *weight*, not volume!

## Ingredients:

- ½ oz. bladderwrack
- ½ oz. oatstraw
- ½ oz. Eleuthero
- ½ oz. ashwagandha
- 10 oz. 100-proof vodka

*Step 1:* Weigh all the herbs carefully to ensure you have the correct amount. Do *not* use volume measurements!

*Step 2:* Add all the herbs to a quart-sized glass jar.

*Step 3:* Cover the herbs with 100-proof vodka.

*Step 4:* Shake gently or swirl to get all the herbs wet and screw on a lid.

*Step 5:* Allow the tincture to sit for 6 weeks.

*Step 6:* Strain the tincture through cheesecloth, squeezing to remove all the liquid. Store in a glass jar (ideally brown).

*Use:* Start with 2 – 3 drops per day and work up until symptoms begin to abate. Average dose is around 20 – 30 drops per day, but some need much less. Reduce the dose if you notice rapid weight loss, (new) difficulty sleeping, etc. Best if mixed in water, and you can let it sit out for an hour or two so the alcohol evaporates first if you are sensitive. This lasts for 2 – 3 years.

*Caution:* People who are hyperthyroid should not use this. Pregnant women should avoid Eleuthero and ashwagandha. Consult a doctor for a diagnosis if you are unsure if you have hypothyroidism or not, and do not discontinue your medication without a doctor's help.

# Calm Down Tincture

*I*f you struggle from anxiety, or have a child with ADHD, or even insomnia – anything that you might need to "calm down" from (even crazy children with the late afternoon whinies) – this tincture may help.  These herbs help to promote relaxation and soothe frayed nerves.

## Ingredients:

- ½ c. catnip
- ½ c. lemon balm
- ¼ c. passionflower
- ¼ c. skullcap
- 1 c. vegetable glycerin
- 1 c. filtered water

*Step 1:* Add all the dry herbs to a quart-sized glass jar.

*Step 2:* Add the glycerin and water to the jar.

*Step 3:* Cap the jar and shake gently to combine.

*Step 4:* Allow to sit for 6 weeks (or use the Crock Pot method[1] which takes 2 – 3 days).

*Step 5:* Strain through a clean dish towel and store in a glass jar.

*Use:* Take 2 – 4 drops for children or 5 – 10 drops for adults as needed.  This lasts for 6 – 12 months.

*Caution:* Pregnant women should be cautious with catnip and lemon balm (both in the mint family).

---

# Other

# Teething Tincture

For little ones who are teething and miserable, this tincture is a wonderful, safe solution. It contains herbs that are okay for children, and relieves pain and promotes relaxation and sleep – it's much better than over-the-counter options! It also produces no side effects. It can be used in adults who have any sort of oral pain as well.

The use of glycerin means the tincture is alcohol-free, as well as sweet and easy to take.

## Ingredients:

- ½ c. catnip (volume)
- 1 tbsp. whole cloves
- ½ c. vegetable glycerin
- ½ c. filtered water

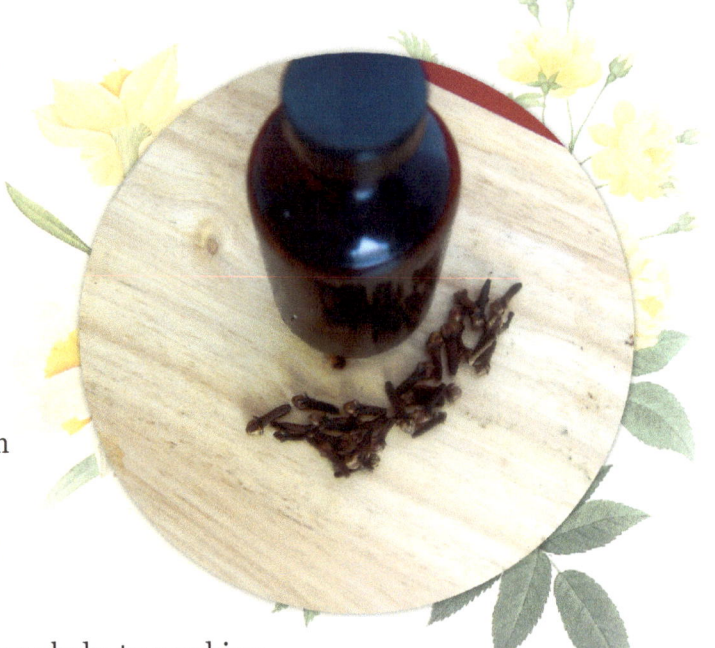

*Step 1:* Place the herbs in a clean glass jar.

*Step 2:* Cover with glycerin and water.

*Step 3:* Place a lid on the jar, then shake to combine.

*Step 4:* Let the tincture sit in a dark place for about 6 weeks. OR use the crockpot method[2] to keep it warm for 2 – 3 days.

*Step 5:* Strain the tincture through a clean dishtowel and store in a glass jar.

*Use:* 2 – 3 drops for babies, or 5 – 10 for adults as needed. Can use straight, or mixed in water. This lasts for 6 – 12 months.

*Caution:* Do not use catnip if you are pregnant – it is in the mint family and may induce contractions.

---

# Magnesium Lotion

These days, a lot of people are magnesium deficient, and many don't know it. (Blood tests aren't very accurate.) Signs of deficiency include headaches, loss of appetite, nausea, restless legs, insomnia, irritability, anxiety, depression, high blood sugar, muscle cramps, vomiting, failure to thrive (in children), and more.

Topical magnesium lotion is one of the best ways to supplement magnesium naturally. It's also safe for babies and young children, as well as pregnant women. We have used it on babies and toddlers who are having trouble sleeping with success. It also soothes sore muscles after exercise and helps headaches. It honestly has many uses and is a staple in our home!

This is simple, requires only a few ingredients, and can be made in less than 15 minutes.

## Ingredients:

- 1/2 c. double-strength magnesium oil (1 c. magnesium chloride flakes + 1/2 c. water)
- 1/2 c. avocado oil*
- 1/2 c. unrefined shea butter
- 2 tbsp. beeswax

*You may sub any other liquid oil (almond, olive, jojoba, etc.) Some have even used coconut, although it produces a harder lotion.

*Step 1:* Heat ½ c. filtered water just hot enough to steam, then add the magnesium flakes and stir or shake in a covered jar until dissolved. You will not use all of it for this recipe, so save some for later.

*Step 2:* In a saucepan over low heat, melt the shea butter and beeswax together, then add the avocado oil.

*Step 3:* Add the melted oils to a blender. At this point, you want the oils and the magnesium oil to be about the same temperature, or just warmer than room temperature. If they are drastically different, they won't form an emulsion.

*Step 4:* Add the magnesium oil to the blender too. Turn it on low at first, then turn it up until the lotion turns thick, white, and opaque.

*Step 5:* Immediately pour the finished lotion into a glass jar – one pint-sized or 4 4-oz. jelly jars. Use a spatula to scrape the lotion out of the blender and into the jar. The lotion is finished!

*Step 6:* Run the blender under hot water, then add soap and blend on high to make cleaning easier.

*Use:* Use 1/8 tsp. for small children and babies, up to 1 tsp. for adults (possibly more for pregnant women) daily or as needed. Spread on a thin-skinned areas. This lasts for 3 – 6 months.

*Caution:* Those with an allergy to latex should not use, or should choose cocoa or mango butter instead of shea butter.

# Liver Pills

One of the greatest supplements out there is liver pills, made from the liver of a grass-fed cow. Make sure the liver you choose is *grass-fed*, because it does make a big difference in nutrition.

Why? They're rich in vitamin A, B vitamins, iron, and much more. They can help fix anemia, lack of energy, and many more symptoms. They're especially wonderful for pregnant and nursing moms, as well as growing children. They're also simple to make.

## Ingredients:

- 1 lb. of liver
- 250 gelatin capsules

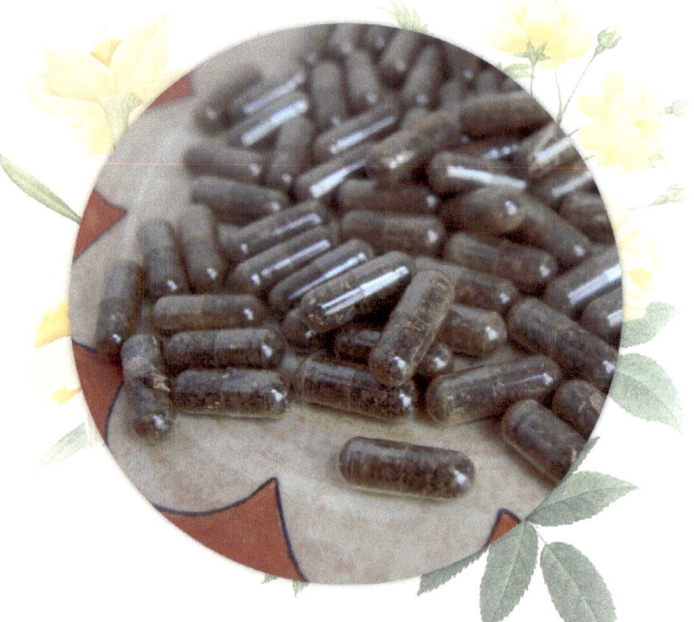

*Step 1:* Slice the liver thinly.

*Step 2:* Place the liver on sheets in a dehydrator, or on wire racks (like cooling racks) on a baking sheet.

*Step 3:* Dehydrate at about 150 – 170 degrees in a dehydrator or an oven overnight, or 12 – 18 hours, until the liver snaps when bent.

*Step 4:* Break the liver into smaller pieces, then use a blender or a spice grinder to grind into a fine powder.

*Step 5:* Use a capsule machine to fill the pills, or fill the larger side and cap with the smaller side by hand.

*Step 6:* Store in a glass jar (this makes about 1 pint-sized jar full) in a cool, dry place.

*Use:* Take 2 – 10 per day. Find your dose by starting with 2 and moving up every few days. When the dose is too much, you may notice reduced appetite or trouble sleeping – back off slightly from this. Some children can chew them if desired. These last for 1 year.

*Caution:* Do not use if you have chronically high iron levels.

www.ingramcontent.com/pod-product-compliance
Lightning Source LLC
Chambersburg PA
CBHW041519280526
45792CB00004B/1305